Alkaline Diet

The Comprehensive Introduction To Ph, Alkaline Foods,
Weight Management Through Health-conscious
Practices, Enhanced Vitality, And The Prophylaxis Of
Degenerative Ailments For Novices

Morgan Wallace

TABLE OF CONTENT

Introduction

Maintaining equilibrium is pivotal for a sound state of physical well-being. The consumption of alkaline or acidic food greatly impacts the physiological state and functioning of vital organs within the human body. The alkaline diet facilitates the establishment of an alkaline milieu within our bodily system. This has the potential to enhance blood pressure regulation, promote optimal bone health, bolster favorable cholesterol levels, enhance cardiovascular wellness, and contribute to various other health benefits. This alkaline diet cookbook is tailored for individuals seeking to attain pH balance, detoxification, enhanced digestion, and immune system bolstering.

1

This comprehensive guide to the Alkaline diet is designed to assist individuals in swiftly restoring, treating, and rejuvenating their overall well-being to achieve optimal health. This culinary guide is specifically designed to alleviate digestive discomfort, enhance immune function, facilitate weight loss, and promote optimal well-being. Commencing a dietary regimen that incorporates alkaline foods may pose a challenge, particularly for individuals who are new to this approach. Through the adoption of this alkaline diet, you will acquire a comprehensive understanding of the intricacies of pH within your body, and how the consumption of alkaline-rich foods can provide not only impeccable nutrition, but also exquisite taste. This alkaline cookbook simplifies the process by providing informative content to facilitate one's initiation.

Consuming nourishing and alkaline foods ensures that your body's chemical equilibrium is maintained, promoting a sense of well-being. When an individual consumes an immoderate amount of acidic food, it can give rise to pronounced symptoms such as persistent fatigue and long-term illness. In this introductory cookbook for the Alkaline diet, the author provides a comprehensive explanation of the alkaline diet, grounded in the principles of nutritional science. The latter part of the book presents a multitude of delectable, groundbreaking, and entirely alkaline recipes, ensuring your enduring enthusiasm for preparing subsequent meals that adhere to alkaline principles.

This comprehensive cookbook on the Alkaline diet encompasses a wide range of meticulously curated recipes for breakfast, lunch, dinner, and various other meals, deftly catering to your appetite and culinary desires. Embark on your path towards improved wellness by utilizing this comprehensive cookbook that focuses on the Alkaline diet. Your physical well-being will be greatly appreciated by your body.

What are the Acceptable Food Choices on the Alkaline Diet?

The Alkaline Diet is alternatively referred to as the Alkaline Ash Diet, Alkaline Acid Diet, or the Acid Alkaline Diet in common parlance.

Medical professionals such as Dr. Robert O. Young, N.D. are advocating for the endorsement of this dietary approach, asserting that foods can be categorized as either alkaline, acid, or neutral based on their respective pH levels.

Broadly speaking, the dietary regimen comprises the consumption of specific citrus fruits, other fruits with low sugar content, vegetables, tubers, nuts, and legumes.

It is advised to refrain from the consumption of grains, dairy products, meat, sugar, alcohol, caffeine, as well as fungi such as mushrooms. It is commonly asserted that the body can sustain a pH level ranging from 7.35 to 7.45 through the consumption of such a dietary regimen. It should be noted that, on the pH scale, 7.00 represents neutrality, whereas any value lower than 7.00 denotes acidity.

Diet And Disease

There exists empirical evidence to suggest that following such a dietary regimen can confer advantages in terms of averting conditions like osteoporosis and other bone-related health concerns. Nevertheless, there is insufficient empirical substantiation to uphold the assertions that an alkaline diet possesses the ability to preclude or ameliorate ailments, including but not limited to cancer, fatigue, obesity, or allergies.

Nonetheless, there exists some evidence indicating that cancer cells exhibit accelerated growth in an acidic environment within a controlled laboratory milieu. Hence, an individual who has a genetic predisposition to or is currently afflicted with this medical condition might consider researching the impact that an alkaline diet has on the physiological state of the body.

Given the substantial increase in the prevalence of these particular ailments, one cannot help but speculate about the potential link to an individual's overall physiological milieu.

It is advisable to conduct a more comprehensive and scientifically rigorous investigation into the Alkaline Diet. Nonetheless, the impartiality of such scientific examination may be compromised from the outset due to bias instilled in a healthcare delivery system centered around pharmaceuticals.

The theory underlying the Alkaline Diet lacks widespread acceptance within the medical community. This has potentially contributed to the prevalence of various severe diseases such as cancer, diabetes, and others reaching epidemic proportions. The alkaline diet, coupled with a physically active lifestyle and low stress levels, warrants additional consideration from the scientific community provided that they can maintain their impartiality.

Diet And Disease

It would be comparatively straightforward to ascertain whether particular indicators such as blood sugar level, blood pressure, cholesterol levels, and an individual's body mass stabilize when their blood pH aligns with the intended range, should this occur. The co-occurrence of these symptoms has become so prevalent in the medical field that it has garnered the designation of Syndrome X.

Considering the prevalence of this syndrome and the straightforwardness of the scientific investigation process, why does the efficacy of the Alkaline Diet remain an enigma?

This might be due to the absence of financial incentives associated with endorsing a particular dietary regimen.

Pharmaceutical companies engage in the testing of new drugs due to the potential for financial gain upon successful market entry. However, as dietary recommendations do not yield any financial gains, it would be the responsibility of academic institutions and governmental agencies to undertake such research.

The presence of a substantial number of these researchers who also hold consultant positions within the pharmaceutical industry has the potential to compromise their impartiality and the reliability of their research outcomes.

Allow me to provide you with a strategy to incorporate more broccoli into your dietary regimen:

I. The vegetable stocks

The utilization of vegetable stock becomes advantageous when it comes to preserving all the vegetable leftovers. We have a tendency to dispose of different components of diverse vegetables, such as leaves, stems, and roots. However, instead of discarding them, we can opt to preserve these parts and utilize them for the purpose of preparing vegetable stock.

This stock is frequently incorporated into soups and noodles as a means of enhancing the nutritional content of these culinary preparations. Introduce entire broccoli stalks into a pot of boiling water, together with the stalks and leaves of other vegetables such as spring onions, red and white onions, cabbages, and cauliflowers. Gently simmer the mixture on low heat, allowing the nutrients to infuse into the water. Please purify this water through a filtration process and preserve it for utilization as a base ingredient in a diverse array of vegetarian and non-vegetarian culinary preparations.

II. Vegetable fry

Broccoli stalks are frequently incorporated into stir-fried dishes, typically alongside a medley of other vegetables such as bell peppers, capsicum broccoli, and cauliflower florets. You may incorporate these stir-fried vegetables into your bowl of prepared quinoa, daliya, khichdi, noodles, etc., or alternatively, enjoy them as a side dish alongside a serving of roasted pigeon breast. The options are virtually limitless.

III. Add them to soups.

Broccoli stalks are frequently incorporated into transparent soups in a similar manner to the inclusion of carrots, peas, sweet corn, and assorted vegetables. Utilize a sincere and finely honed blade to remove all diminutive protrusions from the stem, subsequently dissecting them into small fragments. Merely place them in with your vegetables for simultaneous cooking.

IV. Incorporate them into salads

The raw food movement is gaining momentum, and for those who enjoy salads, enhancing your coleslaw salad with diced broccoli stalks will provide an additional boost of nutrition.
Broccoli stalks are commonly incorporated into both chilled and heated salads. This can be particularly beneficial for individuals who have a preference for consuming uncooked vegetables.

Broccoli stalks are commonly incorporated into vegetable stock, soups, salads, or consumed in their raw state.

V. Prepare them by cooking the florets.

Broccoli stalks are frequently prepared alongside the florets during the steaming process, incorporated within soups, or combined with other vegetables in a mixed vegetable sabzi. While preparing broccoli soup, an option would be to thoroughly blend the stalks and incorporate them into the soup, thus contributing to an enhanced level of nutritional value.

VI. Eat Them Raw

Broccoli stalks are frequently prepared by cleansing and slicing them longitudinally, and subsequently consumed in their raw form accompanied by a dip of preference, akin to the manner in which carrot sticks are consumed. Furthermore, one can finely pulverize the stalks and incorporate them into their vegetable dip or curd raita.

What Is An Alkaline Diet?

As an individual who prioritizes the significance of maintaining a healthy lifestyle, it is likely that you have experimented with a handful of dietary regimens. In the majority of instances, it is probable that the outcomes you anticipated were not fully realized while employing these programs, thus prompting your quest for a superior alternative - one capable of genuinely revitalizing your well-being and aligning it precisely with your desired state. Allow me to convey a notable fact - according to Hippocrates, all ailments originate in the gastrointestinal system. Our physical being constitutes an extraordinary ecological system, and the sustenance we consume shapes and characterizes this system. The impact that food possesses on our health is substantial. It exerts a direct influence on the functionality of our brain, heart, skin, digestion, weight regulation, mood, and overall well-being.

Consumption of specific food items such as processed foods, refined sugar, wheat, and meat results in the production of acids within the human body. This inherent consequence is significantly detrimental and has the potential to induce a multitude of illnesses and medical afflictions. Conversely, certain food items can contribute to an increase in body alkalinity, thereby providing protection against various diseases and medical conditions. Alimentary items with an alkaline nature significantly contribute towards enhancing our cognitive and physiological well-being. Let me explain...

The pH levels serve as a quantitative measurement of the acidity or alkalinity of specific substances. A pH value of 0 is indicative of a fully acidic solution, whereas a pH of 14 represents a fully alkaline solution. A pH value of 7 indicates neutrality. The homogeneity of these levels throughout the entire body is lacking. Certain anatomical components possess higher acidity levels, whereas others exhibit comparably higher alkalinity. The acidity of our stomach is an inherent characteristic. This is considered customary as its primary purpose is to facilitate the process of food digestion. In contrast, urine undergoes alterations as dictated by our dietary intake, thereby impacting the acid levels present within our bloodstream. Therefore, it is of utmost importance to partake in the consumption of foods that possess inherent alkalinity in order to ensure the preservation of stable levels of pH within our blood. Consistent blood pH levels are indicative of enhanced physiological well-being and optimal organ functionality. In addition, it has been scientifically demonstrated that consumption of alkaline foods effectively aids in the prevention of plaque buildup within blood vessels, fortifies skeletal health, mitigates the likelihood of developing kidney stones, inhibits calcium accumulation in urine, alleviates muscle spasms, and provides numerous other advantageous effects.

A study conducted in 2012 and published in the Journal of Environmental Health revealed that maintaining an appropriate pH level in the body through the implementation of a suitable diet holds considerable potential in mitigating various diseases such as hypertension, diabetes, arthritis, vitamin D deficiency, low bone density, and others.

With this being stated, one can grasp the significance that alkaline foods hold within our bodies. However, for all of the aforementioned to occur, it is imperative to fully eradicate any unhealthy, acidic foods from your dietary intake. Due to the potential adverse impact on your gastrointestinal tract as well as your overall well-being, even the consumption of a single highly acidic meal can be consequential.

The majority of individuals hold reservations about this dietary regimen due to a prevailing misconception that a plant-based, alkaline diet lacks the necessary potency to sufficiently supply our bodies with the essential nutrients required for proper physiological functioning. In addition, certain grievances pertain to the flavor profile, as it is often observed that unhealthy foods possess significantly more palatability compared to fruits and vegetables. Therefore, the primary objective of this book is to provide accurate information and enhance your knowledge about these remarkable foods and their potential benefits for your well-being. The recipes featured in this cookbook have been meticulously crafted using selectively sourced ingredients, ensuring optimum nutritional value, while retaining the delightful flavors that you desire. Merely consuming a wide range of food does not guarantee that your body is receiving the essential nutrients it requires. Developing an appropriate diet plan necessitates a certain level of expertise and understanding, which is precisely the service I will provide.

What is alkaline nutrition?

The alkaline diet centers around the consumption of predominantly alkaline foods while minimizing the intake of acidic foods to the greatest extent. An alkaline diet aims to maintain harmonious acid-base equilibrium within the body. This type of nourishment is intended to mitigate the effects of hyperacidity and restore the optimum pH level within the body.

The human body exhibits variations in pH levels across its various regions. Fundamentally, the scale ranges from 1 to 14. Values below 7 are deemed to possess acidity, whereas those exceeding this threshold are regarded as having alkalinity. When assigning a numerical value such as 7, it is possible to characterize it as being of neutral nature.

Could you kindly elaborate on the precise nature of hyperacidity? In the condition of acidosis, there is a perturbation in the equilibrium of acid-base balance. Consequently, it can be inferred that the regions within the body that are intended to be alkaline have deviated from their desired state and instead exhibit an acidic pH level.

For instance, which regions within our bodily system exhibit alkaline characteristics? The blood is an essential constituent of the human body which must maintain an alkaline state at all times. Additionally, it encompasses the lymphatic system, biliary system, connective tissues, and the majority of the small intestine. May I know the regions that exhibit an acidic nature? As an illustration, it is generally necessary for the small intestine and the stomach to maintain an acidic milieu. Due to the physiological requirements of certain bodily regions, the optimal functioning of these areas necessitates an acidic milieu. Consequently, any deviation towards an alkaline imbalance would prove detrimental. As a consequence, the alkaline diet merely strives to achieve a moderate state of equilibrium in the imbalance, namely, to avoid excessive levels.

Hence, an alkaline diet is ideal for promoting the desired alkalinity of all bodily organs and constituents. The diet demonstrates an exceptionally favorable and rejuvenating impact on these organs.

The alkaline diet additionally facilitates the restoration of normal lactic acid production in the stomach, thereby promoting the reestablishment of vital bacterial flora within the large intestine. Due to the aforementioned explanation, it is essential to maintain the appropriate acidic conditions in that particular context.

Distinguishing between chronic hyperacidity and acidosis

Frequently, the subject matter pertaining to hyperacidity solely revolves around the hyperacidity of the bloodstream. However, this assertion is incorrect as hyperacidity could potentially pose a severe risk to one's life, and the human body employs a multitude of mechanisms to prevent such a hazardous occurrence.

The crux of the matter lies in the fact that various regions of the body, namely the connective tissue, small intestine, and lymph, exhibit an excessive level of acidification.

In the event that the blood's pH level were to significantly decrease, it would give rise to a perilous state referred to as acidosis. This particular state may manifest itself in individuals such as diabetics or those suffering from renal insufficiency, and it should be noted that it is a pathological condition completely unrelated to mere acidosis. When faced with acidosis, prompt intervention becomes imperative, as a mere dietary modification falls far short in rectifying the situation. Hence, it is imperative to avoid conflating this acidosis with chronic hyperacidity. So when we talk about the acid-base balance being out of balance, we are talking about chronic hyperacidity and not acidosis. Nevertheless, the prolonged presence of acidosis can give rise to various long-term ailments, underscoring the potential advantages of adopting an alkaline diet.

What are the factors that contribute to the development of chronic hyperacidity?

When we consume a meal, it subsequently undergoes metabolism in our body. Various acids are synthesized within our digestive system and during the process of metabolism, contingent upon the composition of our dietary intake.

However, the body is unable to expel the produced acids at such a rapid rate. The acids should be initially neutralized by utilizing different alkaline minerals. Nevertheless, these minerals typically perform alternate functions within our bodies and are consequentially relinquished in the effort to restore the equilibrium of the acid-base balance.

Naturally, it should be acknowledged that the human body possesses a finite quantity of essential minerals. Consequently, an excess of acidity may result in a deficiency of these vital minerals within the body. If one consumes an acidic meal occasionally, it is not detrimental; however, over time, the body's reserves of minerals required to neutralize these acids progressively diminish. As is often the case, achieving a state of equilibrium holds immense importance in this context as well.

Firstly, we are confronted with a dietary pattern characterized by high acidity, and secondly, a typically deficient mineral content is observed in our diet. Engage in the consumption of a significant amount of processed foods that typically exhibit an acidic nature and display a notable deficiency of crucial vitamins and minerals. This poses a significant challenge to the body's ability to uphold acid-base equilibrium. As a consequence, the gradual depletion of minerals occurs, resulting in a state of deficiency. This gives rise to a range of symptoms, namely alopecia, onychorrhexis, osteoporosis, or atherosclerosis.

In any event, it is imperative for the body to progressively increase its intake of minerals in order to maintain alkalinity in the blood.

The ramifications of persistent hyperacidity

Chronic hyperacidity gives rise to a multitude of diverse repercussions that are highly specific to each individual. Certainly, there exist numerous additional elements in one's life, encompassing physical activity, tobacco use, psychological strain, and numerous other variables. Nevertheless, hyperacidity also plays a significant role. The subsequent illnesses may manifest:

Atherosclerosis (narrowing of the arteries)

High blood pressure

Increasingly poor eyesight

Hair loss

Renal, biliary, and cystic calculi

Co-occurring ailments, like rheumatism

Dermatological issues, such as pigmented lesions associated with aging

Prolonged hyperacidity can also result in a heightened susceptibility to illnesses overall. Inflammatory conditions and influenza-like infections can manifest with greater speed. Furthermore, there is a higher incidence of skin rashes, allergies, and headaches. This phenomenon can be attributed to the accelerated proliferation and enduring presence of bacteria, viruses, fungi, or other harmful microorganisms within the human body, facilitated by an acidic milieu. In the presence of chronic hyperacidity, the immune system exhibits a compromised state of functionality.

In order to mitigate all of these repercussions, the alkaline diet presents a viable solution.

The Health Benefits Of Following An Alkaline Diet

It has been purported that the adoption of an acidic dietary pattern induces the body to extract minerals and essential nutrients such as potassium and calcium from the skeletal structure. This can potentially result in health concerns such as the development of osteoporosis. According to research studies, individuals who increase their intake of alkaline-rich foods have a higher likelihood of mitigating bone and muscle deterioration. The alkaline diet facilitates the maintenance of adequate mineral, vitamin, and nutrient levels in your body fluids, thereby enabling their assimilation by your organs. It is thus advisable for females and minors to adopt the dietary regimen early in life, to ensure their physical readiness for advanced age.

Hormones

The alkaline diet facilitates the restoration of hormonal equilibrium. The primary role in the production of these hormones lies with the kidneys, and the diet functions by triggering stimulation of this vital organ. Growth hormones play a crucial role in maintaining the body, and the alkaline diet facilitates their production and elimination. Consequently, this contributes to the maintenance of numerous essential physiological processes, including the assimilation of vitamin D.

Hypertension

The alkaline diet is specifically formulated with the intention of mitigating the susceptibility to hypertension and stroke. The dietary plan aids in mitigating inflammation, thereby counteracting the development of cardiovascular ailments. In addition, the diet contributes to a reduction in cholesterol levels within the body, consequently preventing the formation of kidney stones. Hypertension has the potential to result in cognitive impairment, a problem that can be effectively addressed through the implementation of the alkaline diet. Adhering to the dietary plan for a minimum duration of 4 weeks is purported to enhance your state of well-being. You will experience enhanced vitality and capacity to engage in a broader range of physical activities.

Arthritis

Arthritis is characterized by the presence of a distressing inflammation within the joints of an individual. This condition may cause significant impairment as it hinders the individual's ability to manipulate their fingers. An effective approach for alleviating the discomfort related to this medical condition is to adopt the alkaline diet. It encourages the ingestion of foods recognized for their joint lubricating properties, thereby counteracting friction. Foods such as nuts and oils can contribute significantly to the maintenance of joint health and provide substantial relief from the pain associated with arthritis and rheumatoid arthritis.

Pain

The alkaline diet facilitates the alleviation of general bodily discomfort. Acidosis is purported to be beneficial in alleviating chronic pain, including but not limited to lower back pain, headaches, and spasms. These may arise as a consequence of an overabundance of acidity within the body. The alkaline diet can effectively counter the acidity in your body and promote a state of neutralization within your systems. According to scientific research, adhering to an alkaline diet for a minimum duration of 4 weeks has shown significant benefits in addressing this matter.

Assimilation of nutrients

Magnesium is a crucial dietary component essential for the synthesis of numerous critical enzymes within the human body. The alkaline diet not only facilitates the release of these enzymes but also aids in their absorption. This contributes to the improvement of cardiovascular health, cognitive function, and overall state of well-being. The ingestion of magnesium can also contribute to the alleviation of symptoms associated with anxiety, headaches, and sleep disorders. Additionally, magnesium plays a crucial role in facilitating the absorption of vitamin D within the body. This vitamin D aids in bolstering the body's immune system.

Risk of developing cancer

Based on empirical research, the alkaline diet has been found to play a crucial role in mitigating the development of carcinogenic cells. These cells have a propensity to undergo self-destruction within an alkaline physiological environment, contrasting with the state of an acidic body. Alkalinity additionally contributes to the mitigation of inflammation and serves as a preventative measure against the occurrence of infections. Therefore, it is of utmost significance to establish an equilibrium and make efforts to sustain an alkaline state within the body. It has been purported that individuals who incorporate a diet abundant in alkaline-rich foods may experience an extended lifespan. This is primarily due to the enhanced capacity of their bodies to limit the occurrence of ailments, consequently heightening the prospects of longevity.

Youthful glow

The majority of foods rich in alkaline content exhibit elevated levels of vitamin C, which plays a crucial role in cellular rejuvenation. Upon the occurrence of cellular rejuvenation, individuals may perceive an increased elasticity and firmness in their skin. In addition, it fosters the cultivation of a distinct radiance, thereby bestowing upon the individual an aura of youthful countenance. The alkaline diet is formulated with the purpose of bolstering skin health and attending to the well-being of hair, nails, and teeth.

This dietary regimen advocates for the ingestion of foods abundant in protein, which are essential for the maintenance of hair, teeth, and nails. The diet effectively mitigates the occurrence of xerostomia, which can pose a significant inconvenience. Through the maintenance of pH equilibrium, one can effectively mitigate dryness and foster oral health. The inclusion of folate in one's dietary intake aids in facilitating an optimal hormone production, thereby contributing to the overall preservation of youthful and radiant appearance.

Optimal body weight

Ensuring the maintenance of an optimal weight throughout your lifetime is of utmost significance. However, executing this task is more challenging than articulating it, particularly when we succumb to the consumption of unhealthy and manufactured food products. To effectively maintain your desired weight, it is advisable to adhere to the alkaline diet. Minimizing the consumption of acidic ingredients while augmenting the intake of alkaline foods can effectively facilitate the maintenance of a desirable body weight. Your body will have the opportunity to attain optimal leptin levels, which are vital for the maintenance of an ideal weight. In order to sustain an optimal weight, it is imperative to adhere to the dietary regimen in perpetuity.

Psychological wellness

The alkaline diet advocates for the enhancement of mental well-being and overall health. Foods that are abundant in omega 3 fatty acids possess the chemical compound DNA, which plays a crucial role in the preservation of cognitive well-being. You will experience heightened levels of activity and energy, alleviating any sensations of lethargy or sluggishness. The dietary regimen additionally enhances cognitive function to a certain degree by promoting heightened activity and increased attentiveness.

Optical well-being

The alkaline diet contributes to the enhancement of optimal eye health. The eyes have a propensity to experience fatigue quite readily, particularly when fixed upon a screen for an extended period of time. Individuals who endure ocular discomfort, including burning sensations and eyelid inflammation, will witness a decrease in symptoms upon adopting an alkaline diet. In addition, this dietary regimen has the capacity to ameliorate intraocular pressure, commonly referred to as glaucoma.

Candidiasis

The alkaline diet impedes the proliferation of yeast infection. This is particularly applicable to athletes, as they have a proclivity for contracting infections in the vicinity of their feet. Incorporating this dietary regimen into your routine will effectively prevent the occurrence of yeast infection. In the event of a rash or breakout, it proves beneficial as well.

Restful slumber

It is claimed that the diet aids in facilitating restful sleep. Based on empirical evidence, individuals who adhered to the alkaline diet exhibited improved sleep quality as compared to those who did not adopt this dietary regimen. When the acidity is balanced, it engenders a state of tranquility and composure in the body, thereby facilitating a restful state during sleep. To ensure the equilibrium of your pH level, it is recommended to consume a small amount of cucumber-infused water prior to resting.

These aforementioned advantages are representative of the alkaline diet, yet it should be noted that these are not the exclusive benefits. There is a wide array of additional options that you can access whenever you adopt the diet.

What Is The Significance Of The Alkaline Diet?

In the preceding chapter, I briefly touched upon a few advantages pertaining to the alkaline diet. Within the confines of this chapter, we shall undertake a thorough examination and meticulous evaluation of the manifold advantages associated with the alkaline diet.

Facilitates Weight Loss

In general, foods that promote alkalinity have inherent anti-inflammatory properties. Therefore, adopting an alkaline diet facilitates the restoration of optimal leptin levels within your body. This implies that you experience a sense of gratification when you consume the requisite number of calories that align with your body's requirements.

Furthermore, it is widely recognized that fruits and vegetables possess alkaline properties. Fruits and vegetables possess a considerable amount of dietary fiber, a proven stimulant of the sensation of fullness. With heightened sensation of fullness, there is no need to indulge in superfluous snacking and intake excessive calories, thus resulting in weight reduction. Additionally, a plethora of vegetables, particularly those dark-green leafy varieties, exhibit a substantial mineral content, such as magnesium, calcium, and potassium, which actively contribute to the process of weight reduction. They are likewise characterized by their low calorie content, which is of paramount importance in the context of weight reduction.

Mitigates the Likelihood of Developing Chronic Illnesses

The optimal functioning of bodily enzymes relies upon a diverse range of minerals. A considerable number of individuals experience a deficiency in essential minerals, such as magnesium. Insufficient magnesium levels can give rise to various issues, including but not limited to anxiety, insomnia, migraines, muscular discomfort, and cardiovascular complications. In addition, this mineral aids in the activation of vitamin D and serves to counteract vitamin D deficiency, consequently enhancing both endocrine function and immune response.

Moreover, fruits and vegetables combat the inflammatory response associated with accelerated aging, while also stimulating the secretion of growth hormone. This aids in combating ailments such as stroke, elevated cholesterol levels, hypertension, and cognitive decline.

Fights Cancer

While there is no explicit association between cancer and dietary acidosis, advocates of this dietary regimen contend that cancer flourishes in an acidic milieu. Moreover, the consumption of highly processed food can result in a dearth of essential minerals, leading to the build-up of harmful pathogens and toxins within the body. Consequently, this weakened immune system makes individuals vulnerable to a range of health issues, including the development of cancer.

Enhances the Restoration of Muscle Mass and Bone Density

Minerals are essential for the development and upkeep of bones and cartilage, with the majority being derived from non-acidic dietary sources. According to scientific research, consumption of whole fruits and leafy green vegetables has been proven to effectively decrease muscle atrophy and enhance skeletal integrity.

Furthermore, the alkaline diet functions by harmonizing the proportions of minerals, such as phosphate, magnesium, and calcium. This enhances the assimilation of vitamin D and the production of growth hormones, thereby impeding the development of chronic ailments such as sarcopenia and osteoporosis.

By considering the advantages outlined above, one can ascertain the considerable merits of embracing an alkaline diet, thereby generating an interest in acquiring knowledge pertaining to suitable food choices. The ensuing chapter will center its attention on this matter.

Exploring the alkaline diet:
The alkaline diet, also referred to as the ash diet, derives its name from its intrinsic lack of acidic properties. The underlying principle of this dietary approach stems from the premise that after ingestion, foods are metabolized into either alkaline substances or materials with acidic properties.
The ingested food undergoes a notable transformation within your body whereby it undergoes a complete change as it is reduced into smaller components. The metabolism facilitates the transformation of ingested food substances, enabling efficient digestion.

This entire process is commonly referred to as metabolism, during which food is converted into either alkaline or acidic substances. The consumption of acidic food items results in an acidic chemical reaction within the stomach, causing significant discomfort and distress. When consumed, acidic food undergoes a process of conversion into acid within the stomach, causing the stomach to assume a furnace-like function. The residue emanating from the food ingested by individuals could potentially contain either acidic or alkaline components.

The consumption of food items with high acidity is known to induce significant acid reactions within the body. This implies that the ingestion of acidic foods causes the body to become acidic, whereas the consumption of alkaline foods leads to the body becoming alkaline.

When an individual ingests food items with acidic properties, their bodily resilience diminishes, rendering them more susceptible to ailments and disorders. Conversely, in the event that an individual consumes food products containing alkaline properties, it is conceivable that these substances function as a safeguard for the body, effectively contributing to the enhancement of one's overall health.

When consuming food items with an alkaline base, your body assimilates calcium and potassium, whereas the consumption of acidic food items leads to an accumulation of sulfur in the body.

Numerous food items can be classified as acidic, including fish and meat, while others can be categorized as alkaline, such as vegetables and fruits. However, there do exist food items that are considered neutral, meaning they have neither excessive acidity nor alkalinity. This includes substances such as fats and sugars.

Therefore, should you come into possession of acidic food items, it is likely that you may be confronted with the affliction of acidity. However, incorporating alkaline food items into your daily dietary routine will effectively bolster the alkaline protective barrier surrounding your body.

The pH value:

The pH level of the diet you consume holds significance in relation to the alkaline-based diet. Acquiring an understanding of the significance underlying the pH value is of significant importance, and it is imperative to bear this in mind when endeavoring to adhere to an alkaline diet.

Determining the pH value of a food item that you are consuming is a straightforward task, as it solely provides information regarding the acidity and alkalinity levels present. Fundamentally, the pH scale begins at 0 and culminates at 14. Within the range of 0 to 7, the substance exhibits acidity, whereas within the range of 7 to 10, it demonstrates neutrality. Nonetheless, the pH level becomes alkaline once it exceeds a value of 10. The pH of an individual's body can be easily determined by conducting a urine test, rendering the process of assessing pH levels a straightforward endeavor.

The impact of pH on your blood acidity levels:

If one holds the belief that consuming a specific type of food possesses the capability to alter the pH level of one's blood, it is an erroneous assumption. The consumption of acidic and alkaline food items does not exert an impact on the pH level of the blood; rather, it influences the pH of the urine. Therefore, when consuming items with acidic properties in the future, it is important to recognize that they will not impact the pH level of blood but rather alter the pH value of urine.

The Final Word
The alkaline diet undoubtedly yields numerous beneficial outcomes for the human body. If red meat consumption is sustained for a full month, an acidic reaction may manifest in the stomach, resulting in a sensation of discomfort. Adopting the alkaline diet and incorporating a variety of vegetables and fruits into your meals facilitates the transformation of your ailing body into a state of optimal health.

What Does An Alkaline Ph Level In The Body Signify?

The positive state of an individual's internal pH can be defined as having an alkaline body pH. The pH level or hydrogen ion concentration in the human body significantly impacts its chemistry and overall well-being. The pH level of the human body should ideally maintain a slightly alkaline state, approximately at a measurement of 7.3 on the Acid/Alkaline scale ranging from 0 to 14. Not meeting the presumed optimal level typically signifies that the individual's internal environment is characterized by toxicity.

What are the methods for achieving optimal body alkalinity?
Our daily dietary patterns, the environment in which we reside, the medications we consume (both prescribed and over-the-counter), limited physical activity, and stress all contribute to the modification of our

internal pH to varying degrees. If an individual consistently follows a balanced alkaline diet composed of fresh fruits, vegetables, almonds, kelp, and cayenne pepper, while also managing stress levels and engaging in regular physical activity, their pH level will be maintained in an alkaline state. However, it should be noted that if an individual experiences high levels of stress, engages in minimal physical activity, and consistently consumes a diet consisting of soda, sugary items, processed foods, alcohol, and other acidic food items, their pH level will undoubtedly be negatively impacted.

The advantages posed by a body with an alkaline pH level
Diseases thrive best within an acidic physiological environment. Fungi and bacteria leverage this environment to proliferate and cause significant damage. An individual with an excessively acidic constitution is frequently weak, lacking in vitality, and typically experiences pronounced symptoms. Furthermore,

they are highly susceptible to various ailments and diseases. Manifestations such as muscular contractions, hypersensitivity reactions, diminished bone density, and neoplastic conditions are frequently associated with an environment characterized by acidity. Consequently, the advantages of a body with alkaline pH levels would imply the exact inverse. A body with an alkaline pH level exhibits robust health and resilience, often demonstrating heightened immunity and a rapid recovery rate from various maladies and afflictions.

What are the steps to uphold a balanced alkaline pH level in the body?
In order to maintain the ideal level, it is necessary to regulate the alkaline body pH through various means.
• The initial step to accomplishing this is to ascertain precisely where you stand on the PH scale. This measurement is determined through one of two methods, either via analysis of a first morning urine sample or a saliva

sample, employing PH tape or a PH meter as assistance.

Have you ever been acquainted with alkaline diet foods? If you have not done so already, it is imperative that you do so promptly. The current generation is experiencing a high prevalence of acidity and heartburn, as a result of the combined effects of work stress, household responsibilities, and the challenges of maintaining personal and professional relationships. There appears to be a significant prevalence of individuals experiencing gastric issues, indigestion, and acid reflux. The aforementioned outcome is a result of the disruption in the acid-alkaline pH equilibrium within the food supply consumed in contemporary times, wherein individuals tend to hastily grab a meal and proceed with their professional obligations. Fast food, carbonated beverages, and similar items are widely consumed by the younger generation, resulting in a deficiency in essential minerals, vitamins, and overall nutritional intake.

Alkaline diets have been determined to be highly advantageous for optimal health. You can effectively manage chronic ailments such as acidity, osteoporosis, and generalized weakness by consuming foods that possess high alkaline content. Alkaline foods hold significance due to the slightly alkaline nature of human blood pH. It is imperative to maintain a higher alkaline pH level in the body rather than an acidic content.

"The consumption of alkaline diet foods offers a myriad of advantages, including:
Improved resistance
Vibrant temperament
Increased Alertness
Robust dental health and skeletal strength
Easy Digestion
In order to maintain the optimal pH levels of blood at a value of 7, it is imperative to consume alkaline diet

foods. Alkaline foods primarily comprise plant-based foods and fresh produce, predominantly consisting of vegetables.

The following is a compilation of the ten most nutritious alkaline foods for optimal health benefits:

Leafy Vegetables - Spinach, known for its numerous advantages, has been proven to possess a wealth of benefits and exhibits a high alkalinity level. It may be consumed in its raw state or cooked with comparable efficacy. Additional verdant vegetables like lettuce, fenugreek leaves, basil, etc. Furthermore, they are highly beneficial as alkaline foods. In addition, they possess a plethora of minerals and vitamins, which serves as an added benefit.

Cucumber - When consumed in its raw state, cucumber not only possesses a non-existent calorie count, but it also exhibits a pronounced alkaline nature. It is highly flavorful and possesses a multitude of nutritional advantages.

Cucumber enhances gastrointestinal function and is conducive to maintaining the vitality and radiance of the skin. It comprises health-enhancing alkaline water that facilitates the elimination of undesired toxins from the body.

The banana is regarded as a complete dietary source, owing to its numerous nutritional benefits. It provides immediate energy and is highly alkaline. Indeed, individuals afflicted with severe acidic ailments can experience remarkable relief from the distressing sensations of burning and indigestion through the adoption of a banana-based dietary regimen. Bananas possess a significant amount of nutritious sugars and can be consumed by individuals without regard to their health condition.

Celery is a highly palatable alkaline food known for its potential to aid in maintaining a pH level within the desired range of 7. This green vegetable offers considerable benefits in supporting your overall pH balance. When cooked to medium-rare, it offers optimal nutritional value and can also be enjoyed as a freshly prepared salad.

Broccoli is consistently regarded as one of the utmost nourishing and alkaline food choices due to its consistent track record. It is readily assimilable and serves as an abundant reservoir of essential minerals such as carotene and calcium. These minerals contribute to enhancing immunity and effectively combating diseases.

Avocado - This remarkable fruit serves as a plentiful reservoir of alkaline sustenance and exerts a comprehensive positive influence on the preservation of optimal well-being. Consuming avocado enhances hemoglobin levels and has significant therapeutic properties in the restoration of homeostasis in individuals affected by illness.

Capsicum, formally referred to as bell pepper, possesses abundant antioxidant properties that render it beneficial when consumed either cooked or raw. It possesses not only substantial alkaline and nutritional properties, but also imparts a delectable taste to any culinary preparations infused with capsicum for flavor.

Potato Skin - Despite the acidic nature of potatoes, the peel of a potato contains a considerable amount of alkaline components. Raw potato juice has been proven to be highly beneficial in reducing gastric acidity levels.

Soybeans - Both soybeans and soy milk possess significant alkalinity, rendering them highly suitable for incorporating into one's diet as nutritionally alkaline food options.

Chilled Milk - Chilled milk has been found to possess elevated alkaline levels and is frequently advised for alleviating heartburn and acid reflux conditions.

Acidic Imbalance Symptoms

Devoting oneself strictly to an alkaline diet constitutes the fundamental practice for enhancing one's well-being in the presence of an imbalanced acidic or alkaline state. In order for proper functioning, it is crucial that your blood maintains a precise equilibrium between alkaline compounds of a basic nature and acid. Even minor alterations in these compounds can lead to severe consequences for your vital organs.

When an individual's blood acid level reaches an elevated state, it prompts the occurrence of a medical condition known as acidosis. However, should it be excessively alkaline, you would develop a condition known as alkalosis. Both of these conditions indicate an adverse acidic discrepancy. Furthermore, the ensuing are also indicative symptoms of an acidic imbalance.

Bone Fractures – Unaddressed acidosis can significantly impair bone health. It is imperative to adhere to an alkaline diet in order to uphold an optimal acid-base equilibrium or pH balance. This equilibrium will provide optimal support to sustain the health of your body and skeletal structure. Please be aware that an imbalance in acidity levels can lead to weakening of the bones, consequently contributing to various bone-related conditions such as fractures. Adhering to an alkaline diet is conducive to fostering enhanced skeletal strength and promoting optimal well-being of the bone structure.

Musculoskeletal Discomfort – Individuals who frequently experience musculoskeletal discomfort may possibly have an imbalance in pH or abnormal acid concentration, exhibiting deviations either towards high or low levels. An excessive concentration of metabolic acids within your system can give rise to the accumulation of free radicals. This has the potential to exacerbate discomfort in the joints and incite persistent inflammation. The level of accumulated free radicals is sufficiently elevated to impede your body's inherent capacity to eliminate them. Adhering to an alkaline diet is the most optimal approach for addressing this particular symptom, as it effectively rectifies any potential acid level discrepancies.

Muscular Exhaustion – In the presence of an acidic imbalance, it is highly probable to experience muscular exhaustion in addition to joint discomfort. Excessive acidity can exert a profound influence on muscular function due to their physiological workings. The functionality of your muscles necessitates the regulation of electrical forces by electrons and protons. In order to facilitate effective regulation, the maintenance of an appropriate pH level or acid equilibrium is of utmost importance. Damages to your muscles can occur as a result of any disruption or disparity in your pH or acidity levels.

This will ultimately result in the onset of muscle fatigue and cramps, muscular soreness, restlessness in the legs, and muscle spasms.

Reproductive challenges – The equilibrium of your internal pH or acid-base levels significantly influences your overall state of well-being. This may ultimately have implications for your fertility. Please be advised that a higher level of acidity within the body can pose challenges for the successful penetration of the egg and sperm. This poses a heightened challenge for their ability to thrive during their journey from the fallopian tube to the uterus. The appropriate pH level or acid equilibrium also significantly affects the viability of sperm.

Additionally, there exist certain conditions and ailments that can be attributed to an excessive acidic dietary intake. If you are encountering any of these ailments, it may be beneficial for you to contemplate adopting a high alkaline diet as a potential means of relieving your symptoms.

Chronic nasal congestion

Cysts in the ovaries and benign cysts in the breast

Decreased immune response leading to a heightened susceptibility to frequent occurrences of cold and flu.

Irritability, nervousness, anxiety

Frequent headaches

Lack of energy

Excessive mucous production

Kidney stones

Insufficient calcium levels, leading to diminished bone strength and increased susceptibility to osteoporosis.

Chronic lower back pain

Maintaining optimal acid-base balance in your body plays a pivotal role in promoting overall well-being, and this is precisely where the alkaline diet can offer substantial advantages. It comprises of alkaline foods or foods that enhance the alkaline balance within your body. In order to preserve the appropriate equilibrium of pH or acid levels within your body, it is imperative to adhere to an alkaline diet comprising of 80% alkaline foods and 20% acid-forming foods.

Herbs, spices, nuts, seeds, beans, and peas are among the types of foods categorized as alkaline. It is advisable to incorporate green vegetables and foods with dark hues into your dietary intake, as the majority of these items possess alkaline-forming properties. An additional suggestion would be to lessen the consumption of food items that are high in protein, sugar, alcohol, tea, coffee, flours, and processed cereals, as they have the tendency to promote acidity. In addition, it is beneficial to consume a concoction of water combined with fifty percent of the juice extracted from a lemon prior to meals and upon awakening. It should be noted that lemon possesses natural alkaline-forming properties, making it beneficial to incorporate into your dietary regimen.

Alkaline Water

One final aspect that should be noted is the adherence of numerous individuals to the belief that the consumption of alkaline water (with a pH level of 9.5 rather than the average pH level of regular water) has certain benefits. Pure water with a pH of 7.0 can be considered healthier according to similar principles as those underlying the alkaline diet. Nevertheless, it is false. Water that is excessively alkaline can have negative ramifications on your well-being and result in imbalances in nutrition.

Should you consume alkaline water consistently, it will effectively neutralize the acidity in your stomach and elevate its alkalinity. Over a prolonged duration, it will detrimentally affect your capacity to properly process nourishment and assimilate essential nutrients and minerals. By reducing the acidity levels in the stomach, this will facilitate the ingress of bacteria and parasites into the small intestine.

In essence, alkaline water does not hold the key to optimal well-being. Do not be deceived by marketing strategies or gimmicks. Rather, consider investing in a high-quality water filtration system for your residential abode. Purified and sanitized water remains the optimal choice for nourishing your body.

Carol Chuang holds the certifications of a Certified Nutrition Specialist and a Metabolic Typing Advisor. She possesses a Master's degree in Nutrition and serves as the founding figure of CC Health Counseling, LLC. Her primary aspiration is to maintain personal well-being while fostering the physical well-being of others. She holds the belief that a crucial element for achieving peak physical well-being lies in adhering to a dietary regimen tailored to each individual's unique bodily constitution. Consuming organic or maintaining a nutritious diet is insufficient to ensure optimal well-being. The fact of the matter is that there is no universally applicable dietary regimen. Our metabolic processes vary, thus necessitating individualized dietary approaches.

Could an Alkaline Diet be Effective in Mitigating the Risk of Osteoporosis?

It can be quite intimidating to receive the news. I regret to inform you, madam. You have osteoporosis\\\". Not a single individual desires to be occupying that seat while receiving such information. Across the entire North American continent, a multitude of women and even men are being made aware of it. The prospect of being unable to derive pleasure from life any longer due to the possibility of experiencing an irreparable fracture is undeniably alarming.

To begin with, this condition appears to have a greater impact on the female and male population of North America compared to other nations. Indeed, in the Asian region, the occurrence of osteoporosis among women is considerably uncommon. "Additional remarkable findings comprise:

It is atypical for an individual's bones to become increasingly brittle as they age. The metabolic processes pertaining to bone ensure the continued strength and durability of our skeletal structure throughout our lifespan.

It should be noted that this is not a condition exclusive to females. "Men are also exhibiting indications of this condition.

It is not solely restricted to the elderly population. An increasing number of younger individuals are being identified with this particular medical condition.

The occurrence of this condition is not attributable to insufficient consumption of calcium.

It is not solely attributable to the impact of decreased estrogen production.

Dr. Brown's book highlights the comprehensive impact of an individual's lifestyle on their bone strength.

Your dietary choices, levels of stress, and physical activity collectively play an integral role in determining the strength of your bones. The conventional SAD diet (Standard American Diet) can be partially attributed to this condition. Furthermore, the absence of physical activity as we age only exacerbates the situation.

So, what can individuals do to prevent themselves from becoming another osteoporosis statistic? Initially, acquaint yourself with the concept of acid-alkaline equilibrium within your physiological system. The consumption of food, the presence of external stressors in our daily lives, and physical stress all contribute to the acidity levels of our body. Of utmost significance, the primary focus lies on the acidity level of our blood. If the acidity of the blood rises to an excessive level, the physiological reactions that transpire within our cells cease to occur. If this approach is carried to its utmost limit, the organism will cease to function. Therefore, in order to mitigate this, the human body employs a mechanism for regulating the level of acidity. It achieves this by utilizing minerals present in acid-buffering capacity, including calcium, magnesium, potassium, sodium, chromium, selenium, and iron.

The primary reservoir of these minerals within our body is located within our skeletal system. As the body endeavors to address an excessively acidic state, it will do so at the expense of our skeletal structure, resulting in inadequate bone density. To mitigate the occurrence of this undesirable outcome and potentially reverse it, it is advisable to contemplate the adoption of an alkaline diet. The majority of green vegetation and young shoots exhibit a high degree of alkalinity. Foods that possess high sugar content, proteins, refined substances, alcoholic beverages, as well as starches, are known to result in acidity. Dr. Brown refers to these substances as antinutrients. The book advises against consuming excessive amounts of protein, decreasing our consumption of caffeine, eliminating sugars and excessive fats from our diet, reducing our intake of salt, and abstaining from alcohol and tobacco products. Subsequently, substitute all of these antinutrients with alkaline foods. This can pose a formidable challenge for certain individuals, with the assurance that upon achieving bodily equilibrium, reverting to former dietary patterns would no longer be a conceivable notion. The satisfaction derived from achieving an acid-alkaline equilibrium will surpass any desires you may anticipate having.

We have been cognizant of the advantages deriving from consistent physical activity for a considerable period.

When paired with an alkaline diet, however, implementing a daily regimen of physical fitness, which includes strength training, can significantly contribute to the prevention of

Option 1: The Alkaline Dietary Program Option 2: The Alkaline-based Food Regimen Option 3: The Alkaline Nutrition Strategy Option 4: The Alkaline Eating Protocol Option 5: The Alkaline Menu Design

The alkaline diet comprises of foods that possess qualities of vitality, vigor, and stamina. To maintain optimal functioning, our bodies necessitate approximately 20% of dietary intake to consist of acid-forming foods.

When these food items undergo adequate digestion alongside alkaline-promoting dietary components, they establish and sustain a state of acid alkaline equilibrium, thereby facilitating the optimal functioning of our bodies.

Once the food undergoes proper digestion, the body effectively assimilates the optimal quantity of nutrients. By proceeding in this manner, we achieve peak performance in all our endeavors.

Nevertheless, in the event that this delicate equilibrium is not attained or upheld, and the acidic substances are not effectively broken down during digestion, an ailment referred to as low-grade or chronic acidosis manifests within the body.

The incorrect pairing of food types typically results in gastrointestinal discomfort. The process of fermentation occurs in carbohydrates comprising starches and sugars, while proteins that are not digested undergo putrefaction.

Consequently, the accumulation of undigested acids in the bloodstream and bodily tissues leads to a depletion of alkaline minerals from various regions of the body, such as the bones and muscles, in an effort to counterbalance the excess acidity. This, in turn, has detrimental implications for our overall well-being.

Consequently, the cells experience a depletion of energy, leading to a compromised immune system, consequentially weakening it and contributing to a depletion of overall health. The immune system experiences a state of debilitation, causing the cells to become acidified and consequently leading to a reduction in their capacity to safeguard our bodies and combat illnesses and diseases in a natural manner.

The muscles, tendons, ligaments, joints, organs, cells, and bones succumb to the impact of various health challenges and afflictions that afflict our existence. We begin to experience nutritional deficiencies, disorders related to joints and bones, complications in the colon and digestive system, impairments to muscles, tendons, and ligaments, along with various other physiological ailments.

Diseases emerge that encompass:

heart diseases

cancer

osteoporosis

stroke

arthritis

digestive problems

ligament damage

The cellular processes essential for sustaining life, such as digestion, toxin elimination, and blood circulation, rely on the availability of oxygen and energy.

However, the acidification within the cells hinders their capacity to execute these vital functions. The internal organs are placed under strain in order to rid the body of its acidic waste.

An alkaline diet possesses the capacity to preserve our bodies from this condition, and, indeed, it has the potential to ameliorate health conditions caused by acid formation. By adhering to an acid alkaline balance diet that includes the appropriate amount of acid-forming foods and a substantial proportion of alkaline foods, you facilitate the natural process of your body's self-alkalinization. The cellular structures are reinforced, thus enhancing the resilience of the immune system.

An adequate immune system coexists with good health, facilitating the body's ability to restore, revitalize, reconstruct, and replenish the nervous system, musculoskeletal structure, and overall physical, mental, and athletic capabilities for optimal performance. The body is capable of performing all of its intended biological functions.

The equilibrium of pH levels within the human body

Foods and beverages can be categorized into acid-forming and alkaline-forming varieties. The pH level is evaluated using a designated scale, and the standard pH value of 7.0 denotes a state of neutrality. In the event that the pH level of any food falls below 7.0, it is considered to possess acidic properties. If the measurement exceeds 7.0, it indicates an alkaline nature.

It is imperative to ascertain your pH level in order to appropriately address and restore balance in the event of acidity by consuming a greater proportion of alkaline foods. One has the option of conducting a pH level test either in the comfort of their own home or in a professional medical setting. This task is straightforward, requiring only pH strips along with either your saliva or urine. Examining salivary samples is the most straightforward approach, typically conducted within a two-hour timeframe following ingestion. To analyze the acidity level of urine, it is advisable to conduct the test promptly after waking up. This can be accomplished by submerging the pH strip into a glass containing your morning urine, followed by observing and comparing the resulting color.

Refer to the provided color scheme described in the accompanying instructions for pH strips in order to determine and consistently monitor your pH level, thereby enabling you to achieve the desired equilibrium between acidity and alkalinity.

The pH strips are available for purchase at pharmacies or specialty stores that cater to health-conscious individuals.

What is the significance of maintaining pH balance?

The maintenance of the pH equilibrium in your body holds significant importance due to the fact that it:

mitigates the occurrence of illnesses and diseases

facilitates the assimilation of essential nutrients

increases body metabolism

energizes you

reduces fatigue

upholds optimal body weight

Hence, it is imperative to assess your pH levels regularly and uphold the appropriate equilibrium. In the event that you are unable to accomplish that, it would be advisable to increase your intake of alkaline-forming foods and continue this practice. The perception that leading a healthy lifestyle incurs significant expenses is largely unfounded.

Consume an ample amount of seasonal fruits and vegetables such as melons and spinach, and incorporate additional items into your alkaline-based dietary regimen. Consume a generous amount of uncooked fruits and vegetables in your diet. Utilize them in the creation of juices and smoothies, as well as in the preparation of salads and side dishes. For optimal nutrient retention, it is advisable to partially steam vegetables such as kale or broccoli prior to cooking.

Methods for pH Regulation

If the outcome of your pH level test reveals a suboptimal value compared to the necessary level for efficient bodily function, the imbalance can be rectified.

One can rectify the imbalance and sustain the natural pH level by:

Consuming a higher quantity of alkaline-based foods.

Monitoring stress

Taking measures to prevent your medications from causing a decrease in your pH level

Avoiding pollution

Adhere to the Alkaline Diet "

In order to preserve your inherent pH equilibrium, it is necessary to adhere to the acid alkaline balance diet. The ideal alkaline diet would entail a composition of 80% alkaline foods. You require a dietary regimen comprising alkaline foods that will elevate your pH level in the event it is relatively low. This will entail consuming a greater quantity of alkaline foods while minimizing the consumption of acid-forming foods.

We have the capacity to categorize the food items in the following manner:

Highest acidic foods

Some of the items included are chocolate, cheese, homogenized milk, wheat and its byproducts, peanuts, walnuts, pasta, pastries, beef, pork, blackberries, cranberries, ice cream, soft drinks, and beer, among various others.

Lower acidic foods

Included in the list are an assortment of items such as coffee, corn, white rice, white and brown sugar, cashews, lima beans, navy beans, pinto beans, oats, lamb, chicken, turkey, potatoes, and rhubarb, amongst various others.

Least acidic foods

Corn oil, renal beans and legumes, plums, processed nectar, eggs, cultured dairy, unsalted dairy spread, and infusion of Camellia sinensis.

Highest alkaline foods

The assortment of items includes lemon, lime, papaya, mango, watermelon, grapefruit, onion, raw spinach, asparagus, broccoli, garlic, herbal teas, and olive oil, among various others.

Lower alkaline foods

Some of the items in the list include apples, almonds, pears, melon, blueberries, okra, green tea, grapes, kiwis, flaxseed oil, zucchini, beet, celery, green beans, squash, lettuce, sweet potato, dates, figs, and maple syrup, among various others.

Least alkaline foods

Among other examples, these items include avocados, oranges, raw honey, bananas, peaches, carrots, cabbage, peas, tofu, amaranth millet, chestnuts, pineapple, quinoa, and ginger tea.

Reduce Stress

Even when consuming appropriate dietary choices, stress can disrupt the body's natural pH equilibrium. Should your pH level be low, it is imperative to engage in stress-reduction techniques.

Check your Medications

Certain medications that you are currently consuming have the potential to induce an acidic shift in the pH balance.

Avoid Pollution

The act of smoking, utilizing plastics for food microwaving purposes, and consuming foods that have been subjected to pesticide or herbicide spraying can have an impact on the acidity levels within your bodily systems.

Results Of Acidification

Regrettably, complete elimination of the acid load in our bodies is unattainable. Acids are prohibited from entering the bloodstream due to the necessary alkalinity that must be maintained by the blood. Therefore, in the event that the acid load rises, it must be subsequently stored. Our adipose tissue can also function as storage sites for acids. The lipid compound responsible for the increase in body weight is commonly referred to as 'free fatty acid'. In chapter 4, we shall delve extensively into the correlation between weight and acid. Irrespective of its storage location, acid gives rise to complications.

The accumulation of acid in adipose tissue and the inability to achieve weight loss are of minimal concern amongst our various issues. The primary concern pertains to the illnesses brought about by acid load. The regions of our anatomy which house acid are subjected to significant peril.

Cancer and acidification

The phenomenon of elevated acidification arises as a consequence of insufficient levels of atmospheric oxygen. This is a rule. In the case where the tissue or fluid displays acidity, it implies that the oxygen content within said tissue or fluid is diminished.

Insufficient oxygen levels in a tissue impede its ability to generate an adequate amount of energy, as the process of energy production necessitates the oxidative combustion of food with oxygen. The cellular structure is incapable of undergoing self-repair and experiencing optimal functionality. In the event of a malfunctioning cellular repair system, the restoration of DNA becomes unfeasible

Dr. Otto Walburg was awarded the esteemed Nobel Prize for his groundbreaking revelation that diminished oxygen levels within tissues constitute a paramount factor in the genesis of cancer. He made the observation that in an oxygen-deprived setting, cancer cells undergo fermentation of sugar, converting it into energy which sustains their viability. In what manner can a cancerous cell carry out this function while a normal cell would perish under conditions of oxygen deprivation?

Cancerous cells are capable of generating energy due to their ability to undergo a process whereby they transition from highly developed human cells to a less differentiated, primitive state resembling that of plant cells. Plants have the capability to generate energy in the absence of oxygen through the utilization of carbon dioxide. Similarly, cancerous cells are capable of generating energy in the absence of oxygen. When the highly developed cells in humans and animals undergo cancerous transformation, they adopt the characteristics of uncomplicated plant cells and acquire the ability to sustain themselves without oxygen through the utilization of sugar. They don't need oxygen. They merely require sugar in order to generate an additional vein, which serves to enhance the supply of sugar.

Following Dr. Walburg's groundbreaking Nobel Prize-winning discovery in 1931, numerous cancer treatments have emerged with the objective of providing cancer cells with abundant oxygen while inhibiting the development of vasculature surrounding tumors. Patients have been administered pharmaceutical interventions that suppress the replication of cancerous cells. Nevertheless, it is curious that the attention has not been directed towards the prevention of acidification, a fundamental catalyst in the development of cancer.

Put simply, this is the modus operandi of the cancer mechanism.

When the accumulation of acid in the body intensifies, cellular structures with elevated acid concentrations undergo deterioration and perish. Typically, this issue does not pose a significant concern, as the deceased cells are regularly replaced. Nevertheless, rather than succumbing to death, certain cells undergo a metamorphosis whereby they assume a primitive state, enabling them to endure and proliferate within this hostile acidic and oxygen-deprived milieu. Such a cell that has undergone transformation exhibits impaired functionality. It has the ability to evade detection by the immune system. It fails to adhere to any directives issued by the cerebral cortex. It can multiply endlessly. It has the capability of inducing transformation in adjacent cells. This entity represents a malignant neoplastic cell.

It appears disheartening, yet their demeanor can be attributed to their previous experiences that have caused them harm. It solely exhibits adaptability for the purpose of survival; indeed, it displays greater intellectual prowess than its counterparts. All of our cellular entities possess an innate inclination towards self-preservation.

Therefore, in the event of an elevated acid load within a cell, the integrity of its DNA structure is compromised. If the cell lacks sufficient energy to facilitate repair, it ultimately succumbs to cell death. Nevertheless, a handful of resilient cells will persist and evade termination.

Contemporary therapeutic approaches for cancer are designed to eradicate malignant cells. Therapies that prioritize the prevention of healthy cells from transforming into cancerous cells are seldom implemented.

Nevertheless, upon examination of individuals in the terminal stage of cancer, it becomes apparent that their acidity levels exceed those of typically healthy individuals. This can be demonstrated through a straightforward urinary or salivary examination. Furthermore, it is pertinent to note that the oxygen saturation level in their tissues would exhibit a significant decline.

Chapter 4: Strategies for Achieving Optimal Results on an Alkaline Diet

Initiating a fresh endeavor towards improving one's health entails considerable challenges. Breaking detrimental dietary patterns can prove to be challenging. Due to this circumstance, it is essential to possess a plethora of recommendations readily available to assist you in seamlessly adapting to your dietary regime and maintaining consistency.

Making the Transition
The process of transitioning from your current dietary habits to the alkaline diet entails a considerable duration. Acknowledging this is important. Should you attempt an abrupt transition, you are increasing the likelihood of encountering failure. It is advisable to commence preparations approximately 30 days ahead of time. This allows for a sufficient amount of time to establish objectives, gradually adjust dietary patterns, and discover a reliable assortment of recipes for acquisition of culinary skills to commence. By implementing a few modifications on a

weekly basis over the course of four weeks, towards the end of the fifth week, adhering to the alkaline diet will become substantially more manageable.

Please bear in mind that by adopting this diet, you are incorporating more nutritious elements into your nutritional intake. In addition to the nutritional content and overall healthfulness, another aspect to consider is the quantity of food that can be consumed. Due to the predominantly plant-based nature of the diet, the foods consumed generally exhibit significantly lower caloric content. Therefore, it is possible to increase meal frequency whilst reducing calorie intake. When engaging in the process of meal planning, it is imperative to take this into account in order to ensure sufficient daily caloric intake.

Commence conducting culinary experiments throughout the duration of your transitional period lasting 30 days. By adhering strictly to the alkaline diet, you will have an abundance of flavorful and easily-preparable meals at your disposal. Currently, if you reside with others and are responsible for preparing meals, it is advisable to request their assistance in evaluating your culinary creations. When the entire family adopts the alkaline diet, it significantly simplifies matters for you.

Commence the task of seeking assistance. The internet is widely regarded as one of the most exceptional avenues for this purpose. Navigate to various social media platforms and commence a search for online communities that are dedicated to the alkaline diet. There are over twelve members who display significant levels of activity. Participate in multiple activities and assess which one or two you derive the greatest pleasure from. Please ensure that you introduce yourself and become fully engaged from the very beginning. You will have the opportunity to connect with other individuals who are new to this diet and can serve as companions for mutual support and accountability. Additionally, there will be experienced individuals who are knowledgeable about the diet, ready to provide guidance and assist you in making informed decisions. Engagement in these organizations can serve as a driving force to sustain your motivation.

Make plans for mistakes. Occasionally slipping up is a natural outcome in your endeavor to fully adopt the alkaline diet. By devising a strategic approach towards rectifying these errors, the overall impact on your dietary regimen will not be detrimental.

Cease considering it as a temporary dietary measure. The alkaline diet entails adopting a long-term lifestyle approach that can be sustained indefinitely. Begin to consider the future and bear in mind that you are making positive transformations to your life. This approach does not simply serve as a quick, temporary solution. You are engaging in something that is highly beneficial for your personal growth.

Effective Dietary Strategies" "Proven Tips for Successful Dieting" "Strategies for Achieving Weight Loss Goals" "Proven Techniques for a Successful Diet" "Effective Approaches for a Successful Diet Regimen

The initial step entails gaining a comprehensive understanding of the alkaline diet. Upon completion of reading this book, you will have successfully achieved this task. Once a comprehensive understanding of this dietary regimen is acquired, adherence becomes more manageable as the underlying rationale for making specific choices becomes clear.

Create logical goals. What is the rationale behind your preference for implementing the alkaline diet? The resolution to this inquiry will determine the objectives you establish. As an illustration, are you interested in augmenting your energy levels, decreasing susceptibility to illness, or achieving weight loss objectives? Write these down. When considering objectives that can be quantified, such as the reduction of body weight, it is advisable to deconstruct the task. As an illustration, establish a target for every increment of 10 pounds. As you achieve the significant milestone of losing 10 pounds, it will serve as a catalyst to enhance your motivation. Document your aspirations and place them in a prominent location within your sight. For instance, place them in the refrigerator so that they remain prominently visible throughout the day. It becomes significantly more challenging to overlook or dismiss your goals when they remain consistently visible.

To begin with, it is crucial to ensure the consumption of breakfast in the morning. This facilitates the provision of the necessary energy to kickstart your day. Furthermore, a large majority of individuals experience hunger during the early hours of the day. Failure to address this matter may result in an increased susceptibility to making unfavorable dietary decisions during the late morning hours. In addition, a nutritious breakfast provides a valuable opportunity for a brief respite, allowing approximately 15 minutes of contemplation and preparation for the day ahead. Make the most of this period to diligently ready and relish your culinary selections.

One notable advantage of the alkaline diet is the allowance to consume the three primary meals along with one or two additional snacks on a daily basis. Due to your frequent and somewhat regular eating habits, it becomes significantly more manageable to resist temptation. By refraining from allowing oneself to experience hunger, it becomes effortless to consume appropriate foods in suitable quantities.

The attainment of any effective diet plan relies on the inclusion of abundant quantities of vegetables and fruits in one's dietary regimen. The aforementioned components serve as the foundation of the alkaline diet. These food items are rich in essential nutrients, ensuring optimal nutrition for you. Additionally, they provide a substantial amount of dietary fiber, aiding in the prevention of untimely cravings for food.

Make an effort to engage in regular physical activity. Before commencing any exercise regimen, it is advised to consult with a medical professional, especially if you have not engaged in regular physical activity for an extended period of time. Upon receiving authorization, commence with a gradual pace. As an instance, engage in three 10-minute exercise sessions each day. One must develop their stamina in order to engage in prolonged periods of activity. Ensure that the exercises you engage in provide a sense of enjoyment. As an illustration, should one possess an aversion towards the act of running, it is advised to refrain from engaging in such activity. If you have a deep appreciation for the art of dance, I recommend you amplify melodious tunes and engage in the graceful movements of the body instead. Engaging in cardiovascular exercise is crucial, particularly when endeavoring to achieve weight loss goals. Nevertheless, it is also imperative to focus on enhancing your flexibility and strength.

Water is indispensable for all dietary regimens. An advantage of adhering to the alkaline diet is that water is considered a staple, with many of the commonly consumed foods being rich in this vital element. It is of utmost importance to maintain proper hydration by ensuring sufficient consumption of water on a daily basis. In addition to boosting energy levels, proper hydration serves as a preventative measure against the occurrence of hunger pangs associated with dehydration. Although plain water is highly recommended, the infused water recipes provided in chapter six can also be utilized. These resources will provide you with the knowledge and skills necessary to craft your own all-natural and nutritious infused water beverages.

It is essential to thoroughly examine and analyze the food labels to ensure comprehension. You seek to ascertain the vital nutrients to ensure that your body is adequately nourished. It is imperative to remain attentive to the ingredients as well. Certain food products may create the impression of being nutritious and beneficial for one's well-being. However, upon scrutinizing the list of ingredients, it becomes evident that these particular foods are, indeed, not as wholesome as their packaging might suggest. In general, selecting fresh, unpackaged food items is consistently the optimal decision.

Ensure that the foods to be avoided are not present within your household.

When unhealthy food options are readily available and consistently encountered, the allure and enticement they bring about inevitably pose a challenge, rendering it arduous for an individual. Recall the adage that states when an object is beyond one's visual perception, it also tends to recede from one's mental cognition. This statement holds significant truth, particularly in the context of food. Prior to commencing the adoption of the alkaline diet, conduct an inventory of your kitchen. Eliminate any items that do not adhere to the prescribed parameters of the alkaline diet.

What are the limitations and inefficiencies of contemporary Western dietary patterns?
Per Dr. Kevin Patterson, a globally respected Canadian physician, it has been found that western cuisine is accountable for the deteriorating health and increased obesity prevalence within the western population. He posits that the elevated occurrence of diseases such

as Type II diabetes has surged in tandem with a commensurate upswing in obesity, which can be traced back to the consumption of an inadequate Western diet.

Detrimental Shifts in Dietary Habits in Developed Nations

Throughout the years, there has been a fundamental change in consumption behaviors and inclinations. The majority of individuals presently opt for fast food take-outs, rather than consuming nutritious sources of protein like meat, fish, milk, and vegetables. In light of the aforementioned factors, it is worth noting that the cuisine is reasonably priced, easily accessible, and possesses a palatable quality. Given the contemporary challenges surrounding time management, it is understandable that preparing a nutritious meal may be a formidable task, whereas the option of availing oneself of the services provided by meal delivery establishments may prove to be a more practical solution.

However, their awareness seems to be lacking in understanding the fact that, concealed beneath the alluring appearance and addictive flavor, highly processed food is fundamentally devoid of its inherent nutritional value. The food industry, worth billions of dollars, has deliberately prioritized inflated profits over nutritional considerations.

The development and urbanization of the western regions over the course of several decades have resulted in increased levels of income and enhanced purchasing capacity. Regrettably, this surge in affluence has given rise to the adoption of a "western diet," characterized by an excessive consumption of sugars, oils, meat, and highly refined ingredients. It is a widely known fact that the detrimental health consequences resulting from the high-fat western diet have presently attained epidemic levels.

What precisely constitutes as the Western Diet?

The Western diet can be characterized based on both the components of one's dietary intake and those that are omitted but should ideally be included.

Presented below are a compilation of factual statements that are commonly attributed to diets prevalent in the Western culture.

A significant consumption of industrially processed foods, as well as animal and dairy products

While indulging in a fusion of refined white flour pizza, commercially processed tomato sauce, high-fat melting cheese, and sugary soda might stimulate your palate, it unequivocally lacks nutritional benefits for your wellbeing!

Tomato, cheese, and wheat do not possess inherent harmful properties. Our physiological systems are incapable of effectively processing and assimilating foods that have undergone refining, processing, and hybridization. If one consistently consumes food items that have high levels of salt, sugar, and fats, it is highly probable that the body will eventually confront a significant health catastrophe, occurring potentially sooner rather than later.

Excessive quantities of sodium, saturated fats, and refined carbohydrates

Excessive consumption of beverages with high sugar content, such as carbonated soft drinks, commercially bottled fruit juices, and sports and energy drinks.

Sugars are present undetectably in various food items such as bread, refined corn syrup, industrially processed honey, baked goods, frozen desserts, confections, fruit beverages, and similar products. The list is exceptionally extensive! Consuming excessive amounts of sugar results in an elevated susceptibility to diabetes Type II, obesity, and premature tooth decay.

Insufficient consumption of vegetables and fruits, along with a decreased intake of enzyme-rich foods, particularly those that are raw or fermented.
Fatigue following a lengthy, laborious workday frequently serves as the

101

primary cause for opting out of preparing vegetables and instead choosing fast food options filled with harmful substances. One of the most disheartening characteristics of present-day dietary practices is the diminished presence (or rather, near nonexistence) of fresh produce.

Appears appetizing, yet it is important to bear in mind that appearances can often prove misleading.

Additionally, it is noteworthy to mention that Australia currently holds a position of concern as one of the most obese nations globally. Excessive weight has surpassed tobacco use as the primary instigator of illness and untimely mortality.

In essence, the Western diet is comprised of ingredients that are rich in calories but lacking in essential nutritional value. Our predecessors, who maintained significantly better health, had a carbohydrate consumption of approximately 20-35%, whereas our current dietary patterns involve a considerably higher intake of around 55-60%, nearly twice as much.

Several nutrition experts caution that individuals who do not transition away from the conventional western diet are prone to encountering heightened susceptibility to:

Cerebrovascular accident, cardiovascular disorder, and metabolic disorder

Untimely demise and diminished capacity to withstand illness.

ADHD, depression and anxiety

Preliminary indications of the ageing process encompass reduced reflexive responses and diminished cognitive adeptness.

Please provide an explanation of the Atkins Diet and an overview of any potential adverse effects it may have.

The Atkins diet entails a dietary approach which emphasizes low carbohydrate intake while emphasizing high protein consumption. This prompts the body to rely on its intrinsic fat reserves to sustain its metabolic processes. The dietary regimen is widely recognized for its objective of facilitating individuals in attaining consistent and enduring weight reduction. While it is possible to experience weight loss, the Atkins diet is linked to the occurrence of certain undesirable side effects.

Recurrent urinary urgency and elevated gastric acidity

An instance of this occurrence is seen in the early phases of the Atkins diet, where an increase in urinary frequency is commonly observed. This occurs due to the physiological process of the body metabolizing surplus glycogen reserves housed within the liver. This disruption culminates in the discharge of surplus water, triggering heightened renal activity.

Indeed, the reduction in weight during the initial stages can be attributed to the loss of water. With the combustion of each gram of glycogen in the liver, there is a concomitant elimination of 2 grams of water.

Based on a research study conducted by the University of Texas, it was found that individuals who followed the Atkins diet exhibited a significant rise in urinary acidity levels, serving as a cause for concern. The act of urinating frequently leads to the depletion of significant minerals such as potassium, sodium, and magnesium. Subsequently, the presence of acidic urine typically results in the extraction of crucial calcium from bones, thereby raising the likelihood of developing kidney stones. The depletion of calcium resulting from excessive acidity also gives rise to compromised nerve function, heightened susceptibility to osteoporosis, and an increased propensity for stress fractures.

The depletion of essential minerals frequently leads to symptoms such as vertigo, exhaustion, lightheadedness, and migraines. That's not all. Dysregulated lipid metabolism leads to the synthesis of 'ketones' giving rise to the medical condition known as 'ketosis'.

The excessive production of ketones, which arises from adherence to diets extremely low in carbohydrates, gives rise to chemical imbalances within the bloodstream.

Ketosis is initiated as the liver metabolizes fats, converting them into fatty acids to serve as an energy source for the body.

In conclusion, following a diet that is primarily high in protein and low in carbohydrates can have implications on one's social interactions. Halitosis is caused by the release of ketones in the respiratory system. It is likely that your breath will exhibit an unpleasant aroma reminiscent of alcohol and ill-health.

Before embarking on any dietary regimen, it is imperative to exercise caution when considering diets that involve restriction or exclusion of essential food groups or nutritious elements, such as fruits, vegetables, legumes, whole grains, and the like. It is prudent to adhere to a dietary regimen that fosters the harmonious integration of various food groups and promotes optimal nourishment.

The Detrimental Effects Of A Body Contaminated With Toxins And Excessive Acidity

The individual in question goes by the name of "Steve" and is experiencing discomfort. Being a diabetic, he holds the belief that his health issues stem from insulin resistance. Steve has been reliant on insulin for several years, and throughout this duration, his health has steadily deteriorated.

Upon observing the dietary choices of Steve, we find ourselves unsurprised:

Morning meal: A serving of three pancakes accompanied by syrup, a glass of orange juice, and a side of sausage gravy. The postprandial blood glucose level following this morning's meal measures a staggering 450. Consequently, Steve's insulin requirement should be a minimum of 10 units in response to this substantial surge in blood sugar. The individual exhibits a pH level of 5.8, which falls below the neutral value of 7. Beyond a pH level of 7, the substance exhibits alkaline properties.

Lunch: A Whopper with cheese, accompanied by a selection of condiments, and complemented by a large 44-ounce serving of diet soda. This is further supplemented with a side of onion rings and concluded with a delectable apple pie. Following the aforementioned events, the individual's blood sugar level measures 475, and his pH level stands at 6.0, considerably elevated on the acidity spectrum.

Dining option: KFC chicken dinner (extra crispy), accompanied by a 36 oz. diet soda. The postprandial blood glucose level stands at 375, demonstrating an elevated reading. Additionally, the pH is measured at 6.4, which indicates a persistent high value.

Edibles: low-calorie fizzy beverages, confectionery bars, and Oreos, yet another unfavorable development.

Regrettably, it is a disheartening truth that a significant portion of this sustenance can hardly be deemed as food.

Processed food items and beverages, particularly sugary sodas and artificially sweetened drinks, contain a significant amount of harmful substances that cause the body to function in an excessively acidic condition and impacts its ability to metabolize fats effectively. This phenomenon occurs due to the detrimental impact of toxins on the intracellular regulatory mechanisms responsible for maintaining optimal pH levels, regulating fat metabolism, and managing insulin production.

Presently, Steve is tasked with the responsibility of handling this matter pertaining to his physical well-being, unfortunately, exhibiting inadequate competence in doing so. It is imperative for Steve to undertake a conscientious assessment of his health to mitigate the potential risk of succumbing to a severe cardiac episode or stroke.

Indications of Acidity

In this document, we will examine the signs indicative of acidosis and outline the actions taken by Steve:

➢ Persistent fatigue beyond the usual level of tiredness.

➢ Dyspnea (difficulty or labored breathing). It appears to be difficult to obtain sufficient air.

➢ Experiencing muscular discomfort and spasms while covering relatively small distances on foot.

➢ Gastrointestinal discomfort including indigestion, as well as constipation and diarrhea.

Steve was strongly convinced that his digestive issues were the primary cause of his illness; however, it is evident that he is severely compromising his well-being. An expeditious alteration is deemed requisite. Hence, I proffered the following counsel which he duly heeded:
"

➢ Steve promptly ceased consumption of SUCROSE, a highly noxious compound widely recognized as one of the most detrimental substances to human health (sugar plays a prominent role in nearly all inflammatory processes and poses twice the risk for individuals with diabetes).

➤ Steve initiated a process of detoxification by availing himself of a tincture that I can provide to you (crafted from entirely natural ingredients that can be easily prepared at home).

➤ Steve initiated the replacement of unhealthy dietary options with alkaline foods. For instance, as an alternative to consuming Oreos, Steve has now opted to enjoy the consumption of nuts, specifically almonds, which are classified as a highly nutritious superfood. Additionally, he chooses to partake in them while keeping the outer layer, or skin, of the almonds intact.

➤ Steve improved his health condition to a significant extent by incorporating limes and lemons into his diet without adding any sugar. This is also included within the composition of the detoxifying potency tincture.

➢ In terms of his dietary choices for meals, he commenced replacing processed junk foods with alkaline foods. Gradually, over the span of a month, he substituted inferior dietary selections with superior ones.

The final outcomes were awe-inspiring. Throughout a period of 90 days, Steve achieved the remarkable feat of discontinuing his reliance on insulin, rejuvenating his vitality, shedding nearly 30 pounds, and effectively managing his blood sugar levels.

Chapter Two: The Advantages of an Alkaline Diet on Physical Well-being
Presented below are several significant benefits that can be derived from adhering to the Alkaline Diet:
Assists in the preservation of musculoskeletal integrity: The

significance of diverse mineral compounds within our physiological system has been already underscored. They play a pivotal role in sustaining the structural integrity of our body's skeletal system. Indeed, scientific research has demonstrated that the consumption of a larger quantity of alkaline-rich vegetables and fruits substantially enhances the prevention of age-related deterioration in bone and muscle strength.

The primary manner in which the alkaline diet achieves this outcome is by maintaining equilibrium in the proportion of vital elements necessary for the development of muscles and bones. These minerals encompass magnesium, phosphorous, and calcium. The Alkaline Diet also promotes the utilization of Vitamin D and the production of growth hormones, subsequently enhancing bone density and fortifying the body's defense against various chronic ailments.

Significantly reduces the likelihood of stroke and hypertension: Among the various impacts that an Alkaline Diet has on the body, one of the most powerful is its substantial contribution to mitigating inflammation resulting from elevated growth hormone levels. The outcome entails enhancing cardiovascular well-being, as the body acquires the ability to safeguard itself against an array of issues including the accumulation of high cholesterol, the development of kidney stones, cognitive decline, cerebrovascular accidents, and high blood pressure.

Considerably reduces inflammation and chronic pain: A multitude of studies have substantiated a significant correlation between a meticulously balanced Alkaline Diet and a notable reduction in chronic pain. Extensive research has revealed that chronic acidosis plays a significant role in the manifestation of various issues including muscle spasms, back pain, menstrual symptoms, headaches, joint pain, and inflammation.

According to findings from a research study conducted by a reputable German research institute, it was observed that individuals with chronic pain exhibited significantly favorable outcomes when regularly administered adequate doses of Alkaline supplements over a period of up to four weeks. Indeed, the study substantiated that 76 out of the 82 participants displayed a modest reduction in the body's pain threshold.

Enhances vitamin absorption and reduces magnesium deficiency: Magnesium plays a crucial role in facilitating the optimal functionality of numerous enzymes present in the body, amounting to at least one hundred. The majority of individuals who have encountered magnesium deficiency have reported experiencing substantial cardiac issues, indications of sleeplessness, muscular discomfort, cephalalgia, as well as persistent anxiousness. Given that the Alkaline Diet effectively enhances the body's magnesium levels, it effectively alleviates all of these ramifications. Moreover, it also assists in preventing vitamin D deficiency, thereby bolstering the immune system and optimizing the functioning of the endocrine system.

Enhances the body's overall immune functionality and safeguards against cancer: In instances where the body's cells are lacking essential minerals necessary for efficient waste elimination and oxygen supply, the overall physiological framework of the body can experience detrimental effects. The depletion of minerals impairs the assimilation of vitamins, concurrent with the accumulation of pathogens and toxins within the body during this compromised condition. Scientific studies have demonstrated that there exists a higher occurrence of the apoptosis process, which leads to the elimination of cancer cells, in the human body when it maintains an alkaline internal environment. Furthermore, the transition towards alkalinity is attributed to the modification of electric charges and the subsequent release of distinct protein components. This action is closely associated with the prevention of cancer. The presence of alkalinity within the human body contributes to the reduction of inflammation and diminishes the susceptibility to diseases, including but not limited to cancer. Furthermore, an alkaline diet has the potential to provide enhanced advantages to individuals undergoing chemotherapy.

Aids in weight reduction: The Alkaline Diet involves the avoidance of food items that promote the body's acid production. You are effectively selecting foods that increase alkalinity in the body. You are effectively priming your body to stave off obesity by reducing the concentrations of Leptin within your system. This contributes to the amelioration of nourishment scarcity and augmentation of metabolic capacity for fat oxidation in our body. Indeed, the foods conducive to adhering to the Alkaline Diet are precisely those that possess significant anti-inflammatory properties. Incorporating these foods into your diet aids in regulating Leptin levels, thereby promoting satiety even with minimal caloric intake.

Enhances the body's energy availability: The pH level of the body directly impacts the cellular production and utilization of ATP (Adenosine Triphosphate), the vital compound responsible for supplying the body with energy. In the event that there is an increase in acidity within the internal state of your body, the proper functioning of ATP production may become impaired, subsequently leading to intermittent periods of lethargy. This can be effectively mitigated by the consumption of Alkaline Foods in order to uphold a more elevated pH level.

Enhances oral health: When the acidity in your oral cavity exceeds normal levels, it creates a conducive environment for bacteria to proliferate rapidly, which can compromise the health of your teeth and gums. These bacteria can lead to various complications, including halitosis, periodontal disease, and dental caries. Creating a heightened alkaline environment within the oral cavity facilitates the body's ability to mitigate the probability of occurrences of these aforementioned phenomena.

Retards the aging process: When the cells within your body are exposed to a significantly acidic environment, they commence to deteriorate in their intended functionalities. This hinders the cells' ability to undergo proper self-repair, consequently leading to an expedited process of aging. Furthermore, this issue can be averted through adoption of an Alkaline Diet.

Heightened Sexual Desire: Extensive scientific research has substantiated the direct correlation between acidic body conditions and reduced sexual efficacy. This can be mitigated by opting for foods with alkaline properties, as the establishment of an internal alkaline environment can augment one's sexual performance.

Are you experiencing a surge of enthusiasm and energy? We have not yet completed our task. Allow me to guide you through a selection of crucial recommendations that will facilitate the commencement of your pursuit of an Alkaline Diet.

Advantages And Recommendations Pertaining To The Alkaline Diet

The consumption of pH alkaline drinking water is undeniably imperative in aiding the provision of resources to every system within our body. pH alkaline water could be regarded as a source of optimal well-being for all individuals.

Water helps regulate body temperature and removes acidic waste products from our system. It transports essential oxygen, as well as vital vitamins and minerals, to every single tissue.

Alkaline water effectively relieves the stress on the liver and hepatic system. This aids in stabilizing all of our interconnected body components, while also preventing the occurrence of persistent constipation.

Typically, a considerable number of elderly individuals experience a daily fluid loss of approximately 8 to 10 servings as a result of perspiration, urinary excretion, and bowel movements. It should be adequate to replace the depleted water by pouring in half of the entire pot's volume every 30 minutes.

The precise amount of potable water required is contingent upon factors such as dietary consumption, level of physical exertion, ambient temperature, and potential medication usage.

Alkaline water is enriched with essential minerals, such as calcium, magnesium, sodium, and potassium, in a readily absorbable form by the human body.

Cancer malignancy does not prosper in an environment abundant in oxygen and with alkaline characteristics.

Consumption of alkaline water facilitates the establishment of a favorable pH equilibrium within the body, thereby promoting overall well-being.

Ionized alkaline water contains denser chemical clusters, facilitating enhanced absorption of water and promoting improved hydration of the body.

The utilization of alkaline water to dilute concentrated fruit juices will result in an enhanced flavor profile.

The natural composition and color of green vegetables will be preserved when cooked in alkaline water.

Rice will exhibit increased fluffiness as a result of being boiled in alkaline water.

Alkaline water is highly beneficial for weight management, as it effectively suppresses appetite in the context of a dietary regime.

Consume a minimum of 7 servings of water daily.

Consuming alkaline water is akin to integrating herbal antioxidants into your wellness regimen, thereby bolstering your body's immune system.

Are you among the multitude of individuals endeavoring to adopt a more health-conscious lifestyle? The alkaline diet is a viable choice that is currently being embraced by numerous individuals as a means to cultivate a more health-conscious lifestyle. Numerous alkaline diet protocols can be found across various online sources; however, it is imperative to individuate an approach that resonates with one's personal needs and preferences. There exist numerous methods to integrate this dietary regimen into your everyday life, fostering an immediate improvement in your well-being.

It is imperative to meticulously peruse the comprehensive alkaline diet guidelines and gradually embark upon its principles. The dietary regimen encompasses maintaining adequate hydration, administering supplements as deemed appropriate, and integrating a diverse assortment of wholesome alkaline foods into your daily nutritional intake. Attempting to implement this change in its entirety at once is likely to result in failure; therefore, it is advisable to proceed gradually. This represents the adoption of a new way of life that will result in personal improvement, a process that requires patience and dedication.

You have demonstrated your commitment to adopting healthy eating habits by taking the initial stride. While it may initially appear to be a significant undertaking or a seemingly insurmountable challenge, as one becomes accustomed to consuming more nutritious food options, the process will gradually become more manageable.

One will derive pleasure from experiencing improved well-being, and a significant number of individuals tend to perceive that the processed foods they previously consumed possess excessive richness or an overly artificial taste. A considerable number of individuals find it unthinkable to revert to their previous dietary habits and express astonishment at the notable improvements in their well-being when consuming nutritious, organic foods. Conduct an in-depth examination of the alkaline diet principles, gradually integrate the dietary changes into your routine, maintain consistency, and experience the awe-inspiring transformation towards a healthier and improved version of yourself.

CHAPTER THREE
The Impact of an Alkaline Diet on Cancer

Due to the widespread occurrence of cancer in recent years, significant progress has been achieved in understanding the origins of cancer, its growth mechanisms within the body, and the efficacy of an alkaline diet and cancer regimen. The stipulation of cancer facilitates the patient to exert a certain degree of authority in both the prevention and combat of cancerous cells. By adhering to a predominantly alkaline diet, this effectively diminishes and suppresses the generation of cancer and other ailments. Due to this phenomenon, it has been discovered that adhering to an alkaline diet can effectively mitigate the onset of illnesses, whereas the consumption of an acidic diet promotes the proliferation of diseases and cancerous cells.

When one considers the definition of cancer in a simplistic manner, it can be described as an aberrant cellular entity. This aberrant cell possesses the ability to solely replicate as abnormal cells. Given that the human body generates many thousands of cells on a daily basis, the solution lies in impeding such reproduction. The most effective strategy, therefore, resides in adopting a proactive approach, which precisely describes the function of an alkaline diet - supplying nourishment to healthy cells, thereby depriving the disease of its resources.

The sustenance ingested by the organism typically falls within two classifications - those that generate an acidic milieu and those that give rise to an alkaline milieu. If you are consuming a substantial amount of medications, this may lead to a shift towards acidity in your system. However, this can be mitigated by increasing your intake of alkaline-producing foods.

An alkaline diet primarily consists of foods that have an alkaline-producing effect, aiming to achieve a pH level of approximately 7.4. If one conducts an online search, they can find charts displaying the alkaline and acidic properties of various foods. If you are initiating the adherence to this dietary regimen, we advise duplicating the aforementioned chart and keeping it in your possession for reference while engaging in shopping activities or dining out.

The consumption of processed foods, fast foods prepared with trans fats, food products containing white sugar or white flour, as well as all edibles containing artificial additives and steroids should generally be avoided. These food items have the capability to support the growth of cancer cells. If the aforementioned content constitutes the composition of your current dietary intake, I would recommend consulting the list of alkaline foods in order to ascertain the appropriate food items to incorporate into your diet at present.

Alkaline-producing food items encompass vegetables, seeds, a majority of fruits, brown rice, other grains, and fish. These food items can be combined according to your personal preferences, constituting approximately 80% of your total dietary intake. The remaining 20% can consist of acidic-producing foods, which should not be regarded as entirely detrimental. Acidic foods examples include whole grain breads, lean meats, milk and dairy products, butter, and eggs. By following this composition, one can achieve a fully alkaline diet.

To effectively observe the pH levels subsequent to commencing an alkaline diet and a cancer-fighting regimen, it is advisable to procure pH strips or litmus paper from a reputable health food establishment. A color chart will be provided for the purpose of determining your blood's pH level. In the context of an alkaline system, it is recommended that the pH level falls within the range of 7.2 to 7.8. Given the unique nature of individuals, it is advisable to conduct daily pH level assessments at the outset. Subsequently, proceed to conduct weekly inspections. To augment your pH level, it is advisable to consume a greater quantity of alkaline foods and incorporate green supplements into your diet. Adopting an alkaline diet can serve as a natural preventive measure against disease.

Alkaline batteries are most famously recognized for their ability to generate energy, thus enjoying a close association with the term 'alkaline'. The aforementioned energy-generating properties have been seamlessly incorporated into a dietary principle. The alkalizing diet is additionally referred to by several other designations, such as the ash diet, acid alkaline diet, and alkaline acid diet. It involves the strategic consumption of foods that produce an ash residue, thereby initiating a process akin to the catabolism of foods. Catabolism, or the process of catabolizing, is a method by which molecules are decomposed into basic waste components, thereby generating energy.

Although the diet may appear intricate, it is actually quite straightforward. Alkalizing diets adhere to modest guidelines, including the incorporation of various fresh citrus fruits, legumes, vegetables, tubers, nuts, and almost no sugar-laden fruits. Nearly all of the food that is ingested and digested, upon release into the bloodstream, undergoes a process of conversion either into acids or alkaline substances. Exceptions to the alkalizing diet include fungi, sugars, caffeine, alcohol, and the avoidance of grains. The rationale behind this anomaly lies in the fact that these food items, upon digestion, undergo a transformation into acidic substances.

The objective of this dietary regimen is to support the preservation of the body's inherent pH equilibrium, which typically ranges between 7.35 and 7.45. This technique guarantees a consistent alkalinity level in the bloodstream while minimizing the strain on the body's acid-base regulators.

Notwithstanding the body's inherent ability to regulate its pH level independent of this dietary intervention, our physiological system inherently ensures its maintenance at a reasonably respectable level that can be easily improved or deteriorate. The alkaline diet is crucial as it offers the body an alternative supply of minerals such as calcium derived from the skeletal system, rather than depleting these reserves.

As individuals experience the aging process, the pH level tends to easily fluctuate, potentially leading to a decline in renal functions. Adopting the alkaline diet assists in preserving the necessary balance required to prevent such future health deterioration. Supporters of an alkalizing diet argue that the consumption of high acid-producing foods can easily disturb the inherent equilibrium and consequently result in a deficiency of vital minerals such as magnesium, potassium, sodium, and calcium as the body seeks to reinstate its balance. Some practitioners ascribe this erratic behavior to the etiology of illnesses.

Headaches, nasal congestion, lack of vitality or fatigue, apprehension, irritability, excessive mucus production, restlessness, formations of cysts, persistent respiratory infections are indications that adherents of an alkalizing dietary regimen would ascribe to an individual with an unsettled alkaline equilibrium. The practice of this diet remains uncommon, as many healthcare professionals are skeptical about the complete benefits of reducing the intake of acid-containing foods, such as meats, salts, refined grains, and dairy products, and increasing the consumption of an alkaline diet.

In addition, it should be noted that medical professionals also express uncertainty regarding the assertion made by proponents of the alkaline diet that acids in one's diet are the primary catalysts for chronic illnesses. It has been empirically demonstrated that alkalizing diets effectively reduce the likelihood of developing osteoporosis, age-related muscle wasting, and the accumulation of calcium stones in the kidneys.

A significant number of individuals are experiencing severe health conditions such as cancer, diabetes, liver disease, high blood pressure, and various other ailments. Physicians tend to administer excessive medication, leading to patients developing dependency on these prescribed drugs. Regrettably, the awareness surrounding the Alkaline Acid Diet remains obscure among a larger populace. This particular dietary regimen facilitates the maintenance of an alkaline body composition while effectively regulating the pH levels of your body. This dietary regimen is widely acknowledged for its cancer-fighting properties and significant positive impacts on overall health.

Have you ever pondered the reason behind the heart's resistance to developing cancer? The heart may eventually succumb to cancer originating from any other region of the body, albeit the term 'cardiac cancer' is seldom encountered in medical discourse. This is because the heart is never susceptible to cancer. The Alkaline diet is arguably the sole enduring method to proactively mitigate and eradicate cancer.

Let us ascertain the etiology of cancer and explore the preventative effects of an alkaline diet. Every individual cell within our organism ensures the intake of oxygen, nutrients, and glucose, while simultaneously expelling harmful toxins. These cells are safeguarded by the immune system. As the body becomes acidic, the toxins overpower the immune system and diminish the cell's ability to assimilate oxygen, consequently leading to fermentation. This particular cell becomes afflicted with cancer and becomes lost.

Can cancer be prevented and treated by following a diet that is low in acidity and high in alkalinity? Cancer cells remain inactive within a pH of 7.4, however, as the body becomes more alkaline and the pH level increases to 8.4, these malignant cells experience apoptosis. The resolution to cancer can be found within the realm of an exceptionally alkaline diet. By adopting a proper dietary regimen that promotes a significantly elevated alkaline state, the cancer cells are unable to survive in such an environment and undergo cellular death.

Cancer cells, due to their anaerobic nature, are unable to survive in the presence of oxygen. They are capable of thriving only in environments characterized by extremely low levels of oxygen. When the body's pH is upheld through the consumption of an alkaline diet, the body's immune system remains robust. This results in the cells receiving adequate oxygen and eliminating their toxic waste. Cancer shall not prosper nor come into existence under such circumstances.

What mechanisms does an alkaline diet utilize in order to mitigate the risk of cancer? This form of dietary pattern results in an elevated alkaline pH level within the body. The elevated alkaline pH of the body leads to the presence of alkaline tissues in the body. Alkaline tissues possess twenty times the amount of oxygen compared to acidic tissues.

Cancer cells are not viable in an oxygen-rich environment. If the cells have a high oxygen content, they will effectively inhibit the development of cancer. Hence, whereas an acidic tissue provides an optimal environment for the initiation and proliferation of cancer, an alkaline tissue will effectively eliminate cancer cells.

The consumption of a rich variety of green vegetables and fruits, accompanied by alkaline water, can contribute to the prevention of cancer. In order to achieve optimal alkaline/acidic balance in your body, it is essential to consume foods that possess high alkalizing properties while refraining from consuming acidifying foods.

The incorporation of an alkaline diet yields numerous advantages in combatting various ailments, aside from cancer. Alkaline supplements serve as beneficial means to incorporate alkaline foods into your dietary regimen. The excessive exposure to heat during the cooking process can result in the degradation of nutrients in vegetables. Alkaline supplements ensure that an individual obtains an adequate amount of alkalizing foods on a daily basis. Additionally, alkaline water serves as a viable substitute for regular water. If one desires to achieve a state of being free from cancer, while also fostering optimal health and vitality, adopting an alkaline diet and embracing it as a lifestyle choice would be recommended.